BINGE EATING

Simple and Proven Steps to Take Control, Stop Dieting and Live The Happy Healthy Life You Deserve

© Copyright 2018 - All rights reserved.

The contents of this book may not be reproduced, duplicated or transmitted without direct written permission from the author.

Under no circumstances will any legal responsibility or blame be held against the publisher for any reparation, damages, or monetary loss due to the information herein, either directly or indirectly.

Legal Notice:

This book is copyright protected. This is only for personal use. You cannot amend, distribute, sell, use, quote or paraphrase any part of the content within this book without the consent of the author.

Disclaimer Notice:

Please note the information contained within this document is for educational and entertainment purposes only. Every attempt has been made to provide accurate, up to date and complete, reliable information. No warranties of any kind are expressed or implied. Readers acknowledge that the author is not engaging in the rendering of legal, financial, medical or professional advice. The content of this book has been derived from various sources. Please consult a licensed professional before attempting any techniques outlined in this book.

By reading this document, the reader agrees that under no circumstances is the author responsible for any losses, direct or indirect, which are incurred as a result of the use of information contained within this document, including, but not limited to, —errors, omissions, or inaccuracies.

TABLE OF CONTENTS

Introduction 1

Chapter One: How To Stop Binge Eating 3

Chapter Two: What Binge Eating Type You Have 8

Chapter Three: Get Ready For A Fight 10

Chapter Four: Scientific Reasons For Binge Eating 12

Chapter Five: Binge Eating Myths 15

Chapter Six: Leverage The Power Of Therapy 18

Chapter Seven: Get Loved Ones Into Therapy 21

Chapter Eight: Delay The Binge 23

Chapter Nine: Make A Vision Board 25

Chapter Ten: Keep A Journal 27

Chapter Eleven: Get Busy 30

Chapter Twelve: Watch Your House 32

Chapter Thirteen: Get Ample Sleep 35

Chapter Fourteen: What To Do When A Binge Comes 37

Chapter Fifteen: Take The Power Away From Food 40

Chapter Sixteen: Be More Mindful 43

Chapter Seventeen: Daily Tricks To Help Manage Binge-Eating 46

Chapter Eighteen: Long-Term Binge Eating 49

Chapter Nineteen: Men, Don't Feel Alone 51

Conclusion: The Battle Continues 53

Useful Information 55

Resources 56

INTRODUCTION

If you are a binge-eater, the first thing you must know is that there is absolutely no need to feel guilty about it or be ashamed based on the insensitive reactions of other people around you. First, accept the fact that, like many medical conditions, binge eating is also a disorder that needs to be treated. For example, if you were diagnosed with diabetes, would you feel guilty or ashamed? No, right? The same thing goes for binge eating too.

Instead of treating yourself with disdain, feel self-compassion, which will empower you to find sustainable solutions for your problem. By the way, you are not alone in the world. There are over 17 million people around the globe who are victims of eating disorders.

The paradox in the lives of binge eating sufferers is this; most of them are ashamed of talking openly about their problems, which fuels misconceived, and negative criticism that drives them further into their shells. Not opening up is not just bad in the ordinary sense of the word but also lethal as untreated binge eating disorders can lead to irreparable medical conditions, both at the physical and mental levels.

Therefore, shake off the feeling of guilt and shame, roll up your sleeves, and get down to working it out. The power to bring positivity into your life is in your hands. People in this world are all attuned to finding fault. The best way to handle negative criticism is to ignore it and move on to doing productive things that will help in resolving your problems.

In addition to giving you some useful, simple, easy-to-follow and tried-and-tested tips, this book is aimed at helping you find your internal power and strength. Because when you are in the seat of control, then the negativities of the external world cannot belittle your ability and confidence. This book is full of tips on how you can manage binge eating that is taking control of your life.

This book's intention is to wake up the lion within you so that you rule your life instead of letting problems ruling you. The author is not a professional in the field. However, the tips and suggestions given are all taken from the real-life experiences of sufferers who have achieved success in treating their eating disorders.

The fact that you have chosen to find answers to the puzzles that are tearing your world apart is a reflection of your deep desire to get better and, believe me, you have taken the most difficult but important step to recovery.

The road to recovery might seem like a long and arduous process but, once you have steeled and empowered yourself with the right tools and the right set of professionals and, of course, loved ones, you will notice that you can overcome binge eating challenges slowly but surely.

So, let's get right to it!

CHAPTER ONE: HOW TO STOP BINGE EATING

This chapter works as a comprehensive summary of all the important tips and suggestions mentioned in this book. Before that, you need to understand what binge eating is. At the surface level, binge-eating comes across as a disorder manifested as an irrational and uncontrollable relationship with food, exercise, body image, and weight issues.

Now, that is only the surface level definition. In reality, a binge eating disorder is far more nuanced and difficult to fathom for both the sufferer and his or her loved ones. A person who has not experienced the pain and agony of eating disorders cannot even begin to unravel the psychological undercurrents playing in the mind of the sufferers.

The therapy for eating disorders is not a simple course of antibiotics that runs for a few days, and the problem is solved. The treatment involves a multi-pronged approach starting from seeking professional help and then attacking the problem from different directions to completely eliminate it from the mind and body of the sufferer. And, it's an ongoing process that calls for a complete shift in lifestyle and mindset. So, let's get started on the learning.

Go to Therapy

The critical element to understand your binge eating issue is that wittingly or unwittingly, you are using food as a way to express your identity to the world. Once you recognize that the cause of binge eating lies in your perception of yourself and the expectations you have of the world around you, you will find umpteen solutions on your own.

To be able to change your perspective of life is why you need to go to therapy. Dealing with the same people in your life will not help you see the new perspective that is needed to make positives change in your life. Therapists are professionally trained and qualified to give you an impartial third-person view; a crucial element to begin your journey to success.

Do use the services of professional organizations like NEDA in the US and BEAT in the UK to get help.

Get Loved Ones into Therapy

The power of love can never be underestimated. Your loved ones are the people who know you best; sometimes even better than yourself. Your loved ones will get an impartial view of the problems you are facing through the professional outlook of a therapist which will help them understand that you need help to get through.

Also, while a therapist will help you see things impartially, your loved ones are needed to help through your battle against binge eating that is bound to last a while because love surpasses all. Do not leave your loved ones out of your therapy sessions. You need them.

Delay the Binge

This approach is a highly realistic way to managing your binge eating habit gradually and sustainably. It is impossible to give up binge eating completely on day 1. Instead, each time, you should delay your binge eating by a few minutes.

For example, after making your decision to stop binge eating, the first time you feel the urge to binge, delay it by just 10 minutes, and then give in to the urge. The second time, delay the binge by 12-13 minutes, and by doing this you gradually increase the duration between the feeling of the urge and giving in to the urge.

Make a Vision Board

Visualize yourself one year from now, see where you want to be, and how to want to reach there. Using these mental images create a vision board that is as graphic as you can make. Do you want to start learning a new hobby? To play an instrument? To follow your passion for dance? Complete your education?

Whatever it may be, create images mentally and then transform them into a vision board, and put up this board in a place that you see every day. This vision board should be a constant reminder to yourself about the promise you made to yourself.

Keep a Journal

Every time you feel the urge to binge-eat, in those few minutes of delay, write down how you are feeling. Make detailed notes of your thoughts, feelings and physical symptoms that occur when the urge comes. Make notes of your feelings and thoughts after the binge too. This journal will help you understand the root cause of your eating disorder.

Get Busy

The next time the urge to binge-eat comes, take your mind off the feeling. Get busy, and do something that you like. For example, get out of your room or house and go for a walk. Go get a hairdo or a skin spa. Go play with the kids in the neighborhood. Basically, get busy so your thoughts are not focused on food.

Watch Your House

While it is important not to deny yourself indulgences in small portions to get binge eating urges in check, it is important, especially during the initial days of your battle, not to keep junk foods lying around in your house. Instead, fill your house with plenty of fruit and vegetables so that when you have the binge, you get access only to nutritious foods.

Get Enough Sleep

The lack of sufficient sleep is one of the biggest triggers of stress and anxiety. When you don't rest your body and mind, it will find ways to bring your attention to it. If your lack of sleep is at a severe level, then the body will find severe ways of drawing your attention to this imperative need.

Binge eating could be that severe method used by your body and mind to tell you that you are not sleeping enough. Therefore, ensure you get a good night's restful sleep each day without fail.

When a Binge Comes

When a binge comes, typically it would come slowly, and even as you struggle to keep it in check, you will notice that very soon, the urge is so deep and strong that more often than not you are stuffing food down your throat without even tasting it.

During these times when you realize the oncoming of binge wave, stop for a moment, take a step back, and notice your emotions, physical reactions like increased heart rate, sweaty palms, etc. all of which are typical of a panic attack.

Compare these feelings and thoughts with what happened in the previous urges. When you stop and notice these signs and focus on them without reacting to them, you will slowly find the power to ride the binge wave.

Take the Power Away From Food

Another crucial element you must include in your journal is the list of foods that you crave and consume the most during your binge eating urge. Look at this list, and first, identify and accept the fact that currently, these foods are controlling you; you are not controlling them.

The next step would be to find ways to shift control to yourself. The most effective way of doing this is not to deny what you crave but control the portions you consume so that the craving is satisfied, and you are also not binge eating.

The important thing is not to restrict any kind of food but be mindful of the portion of food you are eating. The goal of overcoming this eating disorder is to eat and indulge yourself in limited amounts

Be More Mindful

Being mindful of your binge eating session will help you take your focus off food. Instead, your mind will be occupied on the taste, texture, flavor and look of the food. Mindful eating also includes chewing slowly and experiencing the joy of eating.

This approach slows down your eating process, and you will realize you are feeling full much earlier than before. Don't deny yourself anything because then you would be so focused on what you are missing that you forget to be mindful of how much you are eating.

You can start implementing the recommendations given in this chapter right away. In fact, you don't need to read any further to make a success of your treatment and recovery. The chapters that follow give you an in-depth analysis of the points mentioned in this all-pervasive chapter.

CHAPTER TWO: WHAT BINGE EATING TYPE YOU HAVE

Identifying and knowing the root causes is the first and the most important step in solving your binge eating problems. A big challenge in treating binge eating issues is that it is difficult to understand the causes which could range from genetics to personality traits to brain biology to cultural ideals.

Whatever be the reason, invariably, eating disorders have a deep-rooted emotional problem that triggered the issue initially, and unwittingly people fall into a dark, seemingly endless abyss. Here are some of the types of binge eating problems that manifest themselves in people. Look at each of them, and identify your category.

Anorexia Nervosa – This is one of the most common types and is generally triggered during adolescence more among girls than boys. People with this type of eating disorder are obsessed about being overweight even if, in reality, they are underweight.

Such people tend to think about food constantly. They keep collecting recipes and hoarding different kinds of food. Anorexia nervosa can manifest in three ways including the binge eating type, the excessive food restricting type, and the purging type.

Bulimia Nervosa – Like anorexia, this type of eating disorder is typically triggered during adolescence or early adulthood, and known to be more prevalent among women than men. People with this type of binge eating disorder tend to consume excessively large quantities of food in short durations, and then purge. People with bulimia are also obsessed about being seen as overweight.

Emotional Eating – This is one of the topmost reasons why people end up on the binge eating radar. Emotional eating also referred to as stress eating is a condition where the affected person uses food to satisfy emotional needs instead of physical hunger.

Reaching out for that tub of ice-cream or that packet of chips or a couple of hamburgers with fries on the side when you are feeling down are typical situations of emotional eating. Using food is the primary coping mechanism to manage your emotions such as depression, anger, loneliness, or boredom is a dangerous thing that takes you into an unhealthy eating cycle.

The worst part of emotional eating is that your emotions are in a far worse state than they were before.

Pica – People affected by this unusual disorder typically have deep cravings to consume non-food substances such as dirt, soil, paper, chalk, hair, cloth, laundry detergent, pebbles, etc. People affected by pica (known to be prevalent among children, pregnant women and the mentally ill) are obviously prone to increased risks of infections, gut injuries, poisoning, etc.

It is important to remember that there are some cultures and religions that have rituals that call for this kind of eating. Such people generally are not diagnosed with pica as they are not obsessed about it, and only do it as part of a religious or cultural ritual.

All these binge eating types make you feel powerless against your irrational but real cravings for food. There is a deep sense of helpless rage, and sadly directly mostly to yourself, right? Don't feel like this. Reach out for help because no matter how powerless you feel, with a bit of effort and patience, you will find the light at the end of the seemingly dark tunnel.

CHAPTER THREE: GET READY FOR A FIGHT

So, now you know what type of binge eating problem you have. Now, you need to open up and speak about this problem instead of ignoring it or pretending it doesn't exist. When you try to hide something, you will feel claustrophobic and cloistered.

And yet, considering the sensitivities and fears that are linked to the topic of binge eating (well, in some places, it is almost a taboo to talk about it), it takes a lot of courage to open up and let people know you need help. Brushing these forbidden-for-discussion subjects under the carpet is easy.

Sufferers are treated with disdain, belittled and mocked even by family members who don't understand the science behind this deadly disease. This taboo on the subject is not just a huge burden for the sufferers but can also prove to be lethal.

You can start with something as simple as asking questions about eating disorders. If the subject is not brought out into the open, you are bound to be caught in the self-perpetuating cycle of unending agony and pain. It is better to treat the subject with a sense of curiosity and a puzzling attitude instead of living in pain.

On the face of it, binge eating might seem like a simple issue concerning weight, image perception, and food relationships. However, in reality, it is far more nuanced and layered than that. It is a reflection of complex and deep-seated psychological processes that take place in the brain of a sufferer.

Sufferers with binge eating disorders are victims desperate for a sense of control and a search for an identity. The complexities involved in this disorders are mind-boggling because the root causes are social, psychological and biological. Therefore, any treatment for the binge eating disorder also has to be multi-pronged attacking from all sides of the complicated spectrum.

It is not just impossible to do this alone but also dangerous to walk the path of recovery by yourself. You are a victim, and you need help to be taken out of the horrible scenario you have become stuck in. A big battle is bound to follow, and you must get ready for the fight.

So, delve deep and find the resolve to talk about it openly. Then, after the initial hesitation and hiccups, you will feel a deep sense of liberation because your burden is not only yours. It is there for the world to see, and the ones who know and understand what you are going through will reach out and help unconditionally.

So, it is time for you to get ready for a fight. It is time for you to stop suffering in silence. It is time for you to raise your voice and seek help. It is time for you to cut through voices of negativity and self-disdain, and find the strength to start a war that you are sure to win, backed by your personal power and strength.

At the end of each chapter, there is a little action plan to help you implement the tips given. Follow the action plan through unfailingly to achieve success in your endeavor.

CHAPTER FOUR: SCIENTIFIC REASONS FOR BINGE EATING

Experts in the scientific community, especially in the field of psychology, agree that binge behaviors of all kinds including eating, shopping, drinking, etc. are typically coping mechanisms of human beings. Binge behaviors are irrational and unhealthy methods of dealing with negative emotions.

Fully-fledged bingeing urges are characterized by feelings of secrecy, powerlessness, social isolation and shame. Once you realize the deep desire to binge eat in private and away from the prying eyes of other people, you need to be on your guard. You need to ask yourself why and seek help.

Currently, binge eating is considered to be the most common compulsive behavioral disorder in adults although experts suggest that 'shopaholism' or the urge to binge-shop is slowly catching up. Reasons for binge eating behaviors can be categorized into three different types:

Psychological – Psychological reasons are the most common triggers of binge eating. This debilitating habit is a method to numb the pain caused by negative feelings such as depression, anxiety, anger, stress, disappointment, etc. For example, depression typically leads to low self-esteem, poor impulse control, body dissatisfaction and difficulty in handling emotions, all of which are perfect reasons to trigger binge eating behaviors.

The worst part is after the bingeing session, sufferers tend to feel guilty for their behavior, which, in turn, triggers another bout of depression leading to another session of binge eating! And so, the unpleasant cycle continues, and the sufferers get stuck in a horrible rut that they can't seem to get out of.

In some cases, binge eating could also be a manifestation of undiagnosed mental illness. A therapist will be able to discern the psychological cause of binge eating behaviors.

Chemical – When we eat excessive sugars, fats, and salts, the brain releases dopamine or the happy hormone, a natural chemical that is known to create a feel-good feeling. When people binge-eat, an increased amount of dopamine is released creating a feeling of 'high.'

A continuous release of dopamine becomes a physical addiction, and sufferers unwittingly end up bingeing and bingeing because they are craving that 'high' rush of happiness.

On the other side of the spectrum, low levels of dopamine are known to result in depression and compulsive behaviors, which again manifest in the form of bingeing habits like overeating.

Additionally, people suffering from anxiety and depression end up binge eating because they are craving for 'rewards' in the form of a dopamine-powered rush of happiness. Stress makes sufferers lose their sense of right perspective and they end up 'prioritizing the nice feelings,' they get from binge eating no matter how fleeting.

Sociocultural – There is a lot of social and cultural pressures that drives our behaviors. There is an excessive emphasis on the way we look, how and what we eat, what constitutes a 'cool' profile, etc., all of which lead to anxiety and pressure on people. Some find it difficult to manage and overcome this kind of stress-laden social and cultural pressure, and unwittingly become victims of bingeing habits, especially overeating.

And finally, an increasing number of scientific experts state that one of the primary causes of bingeing habits is the inability of people to handle difficult emotions, situations and environments. The lack of mindfulness in modern stress-filled life is believed to be a significant contributor to addictive habits such as binge eating. Therefore, the key element to achieving success in overcoming this debilitating habit is to put your mind over matter and lead a mindful life.

CHAPTER FIVE: BINGE EATING MYTHS

Let's break some big myths and misconceptions in the world of binge eating:

Binge eating disorders are no big deal – This is the first and most prevalent myth among the public. Well, binge eating disorders are among the most serious mental problems of the world. They require timely and appropriate help to prevent irreparable physical and mental damage to the sufferers. There is an urgency for professional and medical intervention is most cases of fully-fledged binge eating disorders.

Binge eating is a problem only for overweight people – This idea is completely fictional. There is nothing to stop people of all shapes and sizes being affected by binge eating disorder.

It can start off as an obsession on weight issues, denying the body even basic nutrition to appear 'thin' and 'cool,' and slowly turn around to consuming large quantities of the foods that they originally considered as taboo.

While binge eating can potentially lead to weight gain, it need not necessarily do so. There are types of binge eating wherein the sufferers consume unusually large quantities of food, and then end up purging the entire intake.

In fact, overweight people are at an advantage because they are likely to be diagnosed with the disorder earlier and faster than the ones who don't put on weight and hide their binge eating problems while suffering silently.

Binge eating and overeating are the same conditions – While binge eating and overeating are sometimes used interchangeably, they are distinctly different from each other. Overeating is typically referred to when an individual takes multiple helpings of his or her favorite dishes. Yes, both overeating and binge eating do result in an uncomfortable feeling of fullness.

However, people with binge eating disorder lose control of their actions and behaviors while they are consuming food. When people binge-eat, they are not even choosing their dishes or foods. They simply and uncontrollably consume everything around them and are unable to stop themselves from eating.

A binge eating session almost always ends with an intense feeling of guilt and shame whereas overeating sessions typically end in feeling satiated or maybe a sense of discomfort resulting from feeling excessively full. But, overeating does not usually end with guilt and shame.

Binge eating can be fixed by just choosing to eat less – A complete and ruthless myth spread by insensitive people who have no idea what the sufferers are going through! You cannot 'fix' binge eating by merely changing the quality and quantity of food consumed. It is a complex, nuanced mental disorder in which food has a significant control over the life of the sufferer. It requires significant behavioral changes that need the support and help of professionals and the understanding and care of loved ones.

Binge eating only involves high-fat foods – Binge eating sufferers can end up being controlled by any kind of food, and not just high-fat foods. While most have cravings for certain types of foods, people on a binge eating session can eat even foods they dislike or would never have chosen to consume during normal times.

Binge eating affects only women or adults – This disorder can affect anyone irrespective of caste, creed, age, gender, etc.

So, be wary of these misconceived ideas about binge eating. Knowing the correct facts will help you tackle your problem more objectively than being without the right knowledge.

CHAPTER SIX: LEVERAGE THE POWER OF THERAPY

Nearly all types of binge eating disorders are connected to some unresolved issue within the sufferer's mind. Food is only a coping mechanism that these victims use in the hope that these problems and emotions disappear forever from their systems. This is a futile hope.

The food eaten during the binge eating session seems to soothe the pain giving sufferers false hopes that the problem has gone away. However, binge eating works just like a painkiller, which takes away that feeling of pain for a little while. But, the underlying cause of the agony is still there bubbling away and waiting to erupt and far more ferociously than before.

Similarly, the binge eating mechanism that you use to cope with your pain is not really solving the deep-rooted, underlying cause. So, when the effect of the binge eating wears off, the agony comes back with added vigor filling you with more guilt, shame and sense of worthlessness than you had before.

Going to a therapist will help you identify the actual problem that is represented by your binge eating problem. You then work on that root cause, and not the symptom manifesting through the eating disorder. When the root of the problem is handled, then the symptoms disappear on their own.

A sufferer with all the help of loved ones will not be very successful at finding the core issue that is being manifested as binge eating, and that is why you need to go to therapy. Other immensely useful advantages of seeking professional help include:

- Guided and customized help regarding realistic diet plans, how to identify and track triggers, and how to find alternate coping mechanisms.
- Access to scientifically proven modern-day therapies such cognitive behavioral therapy (CBT) in which you get qualified medical personnel to help you sort out and categorize patterns of thoughts and feelings including the unacknowledged ones that could be the root cause of your binge eating problems.
- Access to approved medication for anxiety/depression, social phobias, and other forms of obsessive-compulsive disorders (OCD)

The following help forums are available for binge eating sufferers:

BEAT – is a help forum for binge eating sufferers in the UK. In this place, you can find professional help in the form of therapists, doctors, psychiatrists, counselors, and nutritionists who can help you identify your problem and formulate customized treatment strategies. You can speak to other sufferers in the various chat rooms, and find some solace in the fact that you are not alone.

NEDA – stands for National Eating Disorders Association is a forum for sufferers in the US, which run support systems similar to BEAT in the UK.

Other online support systems – In addition to the formal associations mentioned above, there are multiple online forums that you can join, and speak to, and seek support to solve your binge eating problems.

The most important thing is to accept and know that you need professional help. It would be naïve to think you can do everything yourself. Binge eating is a serious mental disorder that mandatorily requires professional help and support.

There are people in this world standing by to help you. Don't ignore their voices. Reach out, and take the extended hand, and watch your binge eating problems disappear sooner than later.

Look at the last chapter titled 'Useful Information' in this book, and book an appointment with a service provider immediately.

CHAPTER SEVEN: GET LOVED ONES INTO THERAPY

After you, the people most affected by your binge-eating disorder are your loved ones. Ignorance and lack of understanding drive them crazy as much as the pain of your disorder drives you nuts. Many times, wittingly or unwittingly, loved ones say hurtful things to the sufferer without understanding the depth of the agony that the sufferer undergoes.

Therapy is, therefore, not just for you, the patient, but also for your support system, which typically consists of your loved ones. Here are some reasons why loved ones have to be included in your therapy:

Loved ones need professional guidance as much as you do – Your loved ones are as new to the problems associated with binge eating as much as you are. In fact, they are so hurt at seeing you behave irrationally during your binge eating sessions, that many choose the brushing-under-the-carpet routine to handle their own hurt and pain.

Your loved ones need to understand what you are going through. They need to be told that binge eating disorders are not simple overeating problems. This disorder is a manifestation of deep-seated biological and psychological problems that require professional intervention. A therapist is well-equipped to coach your loved ones, and therefore, they should be included in your therapy.

They can identify and recognize critical signs – Loved ones are still in a learning curve when it comes to recognizing and identifying signs of binge-eating urges and other symptoms. They will learn how to recognize critical signs when they are included in your therapy sessions.

This approach will help you immensely because, during the initial stages of the fight, there are bound to be a lot of occasions where you are unable to control your urges. You will need people to help you manage your feelings and emotions. For this, the concerned people must understand and accept that there is a problem, recognize critical signs, and then help you counter them in various ways.

Discussing your problems will be easier – Family members form the foundation of your support system. You should be able to explain your pain and agony to them. Without the presence of a qualified and impartial therapist, such painful discussions invariably end in misunderstandings and hurtful conversations because both of you lack the scientific knowledge to understand the crux of binge eating disorder.

When you discuss your problems with your loved in the presence of an impartial and trained therapist, he or she acts like a facilitator giving you support in the form of scientific explanations of your emotional pain. This helps in improving the understanding of your issues both by you and your loved ones.

Therapists will have scientifically-backed statistics that help you and your loved ones know that you are not alone. There are many more people out there in the world who are struggling as much as you are.

Therefore, don't hesitate to let your loved ones know you need professional help, and take them along with you for your next therapy session.

CHAPTER EIGHT: DELAY THE BINGE

Delay the binge and don't deny your body and mind their cravings. What happens when you are told by someone not to think of a white elephant? Well, your mind immediately conjures up images of the white elephant, right? The same thing happens when you deny your body its cravings.

These cravings are never forgotten by your body. The more you deny them, the deeper the cravings get, and you are stuck in this perpetual hamster wheel one half of which is the denying part, and the other half is the bingeing part.

The way to break this hamster wheel is to slowly but steadily delay feeding your cravings so that your mind gradually comes to accept the fact that you are, at some point of time, going to eat what you want. This feeling takes the edge off the cravings, and each time you delay your binge, you are blunting its sharpness a little bit. So, here's what you can do:

- You have decided to stop bingeing. Within an hour of your decision, cravings are bound to come. Be ready for them because your body needs time to get accustomed to not getting food any earlier.
- Now, give yourself 10 minutes, and then give in to your craving.
- After you binge-eat, you are going to feel horrible and get into your usual guilt trip. Accept this as part of the healing process.

- Despite feeling horrible earlier, you will get the binge-eating urge again. This time around, wait for 15 minutes before you give in.
- The third time around, give yourself 20 minutes, and so forth.

With this delay, your body and mind are getting slowly but surely accustomed to the fact that you are making efforts to take control of your life. The physical and mental tortures will reduce with each delay, and sooner rather than later, you will find yourself getting better with handling your binge-eating urges.

Yes, there will be times when you feel you cannot wait until the allocated time to give in to your urge. Don't deny yourself beyond a control point because then the risk of falling into that denying and bingeing hamster wheel is high.

Be patient with yourself. If you think it is easier to increase your delay period by 2-3 minutes instead of 5 minutes, please do so. Remember to listen to your body because it knows you best. These are only guidelines to give you an understanding of how these tricks can work on the mind.

The final decision on the nitty-gritty of the strategy should be based on your needs and lifestyle. But, remember delaying the binge a little at a time is bound to give sustainable results instead of trying to stop your binge-eating habit all at once.

It would be like a person weighing 200 pounds who wants to lose 100 pounds within a month. The plan is sure to backfire, right? Any rushed plan to solve a deep-rooted issue will only worsen the situation, and not solve it.

Therefore, take baby steps, and gradually increase the intensity of controlling your binge-eating urges, and you are sure to achieve sustainable success. Start right now with a 5-minute delay of your binge.

CHAPTER NINE: MAKE A VISION BOARD

Vision board ideas are excellent motivational tools to help you achieve your dreams and desires. Create a vision board with details and images of how you see your life panning out with regard to your binge eating issues by the end of this year. Here are some useful tips to help you:

Write down your goals – What do you want to achieve at the end of this year? Do you see yourself completely free from the pains of binge eating? Do you see a happy, healthy persona smiling back at you when you look in the mirror? Do you see yourself achieving your academic and work goals that are being curtailed now because of your binge eating problems? Answer these questions, and make a list of goals you want to achieve.

Pick up old magazines and newspapers with beautiful pictures in them – Collect some old magazines that you are not using anymore. Ask your friends and family members too. Just ensure there are beautiful, colorful, creative, and stunning pictures in them.

Find images that are aligned with your goals – Go through the magazines, and find pictures and images (make sure they are colorful and beautiful) that represent your goals. Identify pictures that speak to you meaningfully. For example, you find something, and you involuntarily say something like, "Yes, this is precisely where I want to be." Cut out these pictures neatly.

For example, if your goal is to graduate from college after overcoming your binge eating problem, then find a picture that represents this idea. It could be a picture of a graduate student or an image of a certificate or something like that. Find plenty of such pictures all aligning with your goals(s).

Create a collage with these pictures – Make a colorful collage with your picture collection. Buy yourself a nice, large-sized poster paper and create your collage on it. Add your goals all around the collage. Feel free to include suitable quotes from your idols and people you admire. Add affirmation sentences too.

Also, make a list of words that reflect how you want to feel when you achieve your goal(s). Write these words all over the collage or in places where the word or phrase fits a particular picture.

Place your vision board where you can see it daily – You must touch base with your vision board on a daily basis to keep reminding yourself of your purpose and goals. Therefore, you must make sure you place your vision board where it is visible to you day in and day out. See it when you wake up, see it when your bingeing urge attacks, see it before you go to bed, and see it whenever you feel low and unhappy.

The visualization of a great future will motivate you to overcome temporary setbacks and help you get back on track. Spend some time every day with your vision board. This vision board should ideally help you create a new and exciting version of yourself. It should help you think of a future self where you are managing all your negative emotions powerfully without even thinking of raiding the fridge. An alternative identity in your mind will drive your real self toward working unfailingly to realize the vision of your virtual reality.

Right now, take a paper and pencil and, in one sentence, write down what will be your final goal at the end of one year. You can build on this one sentence using the tips given in this chapter.

CHAPTER TEN: KEEP A JOURNAL

Journaling is a handy tool in the treatment of binge eating disorders. Writing down something, especially by hand, helps you get an objective view of your thoughts and ideas, and also help you to calm down so that you can think better.

The act of writing forces your mind to slow down so that it works at the same speed as your hand as it makes words on paper. This slowing down of your mind is very useful in managing emotions.

Go ahead, and buy yourself a good diary that matches with your personality. For example, if you like your diary pretty and decorative, then get one like that. If you are a more functional person, who likes to keep things at a minimal, get yourself a simple, elegant diary that has plenty of writing area. Here are some of the things you must include in your journal each day:

Morning thoughts – What were the thoughts going on in your head as soon as you wake up? Did you get a good night's rest? Are you feeling refreshed? What things are you looking forward to today? What things are you dreading today? In addition to these thoughts, write an affirmation that motivates you to meet with the challenges of the day with added vigor.

When a bingeing urge comes on – You must definitely keep a note for this. Can you recognize the triggers for the bingeing urge? Write them down immediately. What are you feeling? What are your emotions? Can you think of an event or episode or comment passed by someone that set off these negative thoughts in your head?

The best part of journaling is that it can help you accomplish the delay-the-binge goal. When you pick up your diary to write down your thoughts, you are automatically delaying the binge by turning the attention of your mind to productive work giving you the required impetus to delay your binge at least until you finish completing your journaling work. Therefore, the more detailed you make your notes, the more time you will spend on the activity, and the more you will be able to delay your binge.

After a bingeing session – After your bingeing session, again write down your feelings, thoughts and what you believe happened when you were engaged in the bingeing activity. Can you recall the foods you consumed? Do you recall where you sat down? Can you recall the emotions that played in your mind while you binged?

Did you focus on one type of food? List down the foods that you ate or whatever you can remember. Are you feeling guilty or ashamed? Write down the reasons for these feelings?

Track your positive thoughts – Don't forget to track your positive thoughts and their triggers as well. You can use them to counter negative thoughts whenever needed. What made you happy or joyful? Write down the triggers so that you can use them when you are feeling down.

End-of-the-day notes – Before retiring for the day, write down your thoughts on how the day went. How many binge eating urges did you have? How many were you able to delay? How did you delay the binge? How often did you fail to delay the binge? Why were you not able to delay the binge? What were the things and events that made you happy? What made you unhappy?

This journal should become your binge eating Bible that you will continuously refer to whenever you are in doubt. For now, go out, and buy a diary for yourself. Write your name and date on the first page. And write down two of the topmost feelings playing in your mind.

CHAPTER ELEVEN: GET BUSY

Find yourself something productive to do. If you don't have a job, then go and find a hobby. Join a creative club of your choice. If you love dancing, then join an aerobics or dance club, and feel your endorphins build up in your system even as your mind is completely off food.

When you get busy with other things, your mind and heart put the right perspective on food. The irrational relationship with food that all sufferers of binge-eating have will be replaced with a healthy relationship with food. You will realize that food is a beautiful element of human life, and it is meant for the enjoyment of human beings, and not to sate a craving that bogs you down. Here are some simple tips to get busy:

Find your passion – Identify what you love doing most, and spend your time and energy productively indulging in that activity. It could be writing, beauty and fashion, painting, music and dancing, or anything else. When you do something you love, you don't have to work a single day, and worry about anxieties and stresses; the critical elements that trigger binge-eating urges.

Join a class and learn something new – It could be a new language or learning to play an instrument or cooking/baking classes or dance classes or anything else that excites you. Meeting new people as you learn new skills will build your confidence level significantly. Confidence is another key item for self-esteem, which is directly connected to binge-eating personalities.

And, if you are a student, then please turn your focus onto your schoolwork, and ensure you do well in class. Get your assignments done regularly, submit your papers on time, read and learn from books recommended by your teachers, and focus your entire attention on schoolwork. Binge-eating will slowly but surely disappear from your life.

Get physical – Go for a walk or run or hit the gym. Getting physical activity not only keeps you fit and healthy but also works as a great stress-reliever.

Surround yourself with friends and family – Unconditional love from your loved one is the biggest asset you have. Don't underestimate its power. Surround yourself with love from such people, and you will find the strength to overcome binge-eating urges.

Speak to them about your problem, and include them in your therapy sessions. Spend quality time with them whenever you can. It's one of the best ways to keep yourself happy and have fun, leaving the gnawing anxieties of binge-eating behind you.

Indulge in relaxation techniques – Yes, it is important to sit back and relax occasionally. Treat yourself to a spa, watch a movie, go shopping or simply lie back and read a favorite book. Just remember not to indulge in something that reminds you of food. For example, if you are a person who munches on something (even as innocuous non-buttered popcorn) while reading a book or watching a movie, then you must be conscious of the fact that your mind could be drawn toward food. Keep this in mind, and relax in ways that are most suitable for you.

CHAPTER TWELVE: WATCH YOUR HOUSE

Suppose a chain smoker is trying to give up smoking, then the first thing he or she should do is to get rid of all the cigarettes lying around in easily accessible places. Similarly, an alcoholic trying to give up drinking should not be given access to liquor at all.

In the same way, you must ensure your house is completely clear of all junk foods so that you simply don't have it within easy reach. If you can ride the binge wave without getting access to junk foods, then it means you are inching towards success.

Avoid keeping the foods that you crave during your binge-eating sessions. You can get a list of this from the journal you keep. In this journal, in addition to writing down feelings and thoughts, make notes about the food you binged on. Make a list of these foods, and ensure your house is free of them.

Here are some more tips on how to keep clear of junk and unhealthy foods from your house:

Start from your kitchen cupboards – It might take you a couple of hours to clear out your kitchen cupboards. Clear them of all junk foods, all processed foods, all refined sugars, etc. Out of sight is out of mind is the best rule to follow in such situations. If you cannot see junk foods, your mind will forget about it.

If you have not been able to ride over the binge wave (which is expected during the initial stages and during the ups and downs), then go to the store, and pick up enough for a small portion for that one binge session only. Like this, you can control your portions if you keep your house clear of foods that trigger binge-eating.

Then, attack your fridge – Remove all the ice-cream, and preservative-rich, sugar-laden, and salt-laden heat-and-eat frozen foods. Remove creams and sauces that are also filled with the wrong ingredients. Remove calorie-filled cheeses. Get rid of everything except perhaps milk and a few nutritive dairy products that are good for your health.

Keep your fridge as empty as you can. If the urge to eat an ice-cream is uncontrollable, then walk to the nearest ice-cream parlor, and get yourself a small-sized cup to manage the urge at that particular point in time.

Always keep something healthy to eat at home – It is natural for most of us to eat what is easy to access. So, during your binge urges, if you have access only to nutritious, healthy foods and snacks, then it is quite likely that you won't even feel like stepping out of your house to buy even single portions of junk food.

It is quite possible that you will simply binge eat on healthy foods which is better than binge eating junk. Therefore, keep healthy snacks easily accessible in your house. Stock your house with plenty of fresh fruit and vegetables. When you have a craving for sugar, eat a piece of fruit, and you could feel satiated.

If you feel like munching on something crunchy, choose carrot juliennes over chips. Make your own fries by baking potatoes instead of frying them.

Make sure your home has plenty of stock of whole grains – Make sure your home is well-stocked with whole grains such as quinoa, brown and unpolished rice, millet, buckwheat, etc. so that when you feel like cooking, you have only these ingredients to use.

So, your first action concerning watching your house is to clear out your cupboards in the kitchen. Take a big bag, and fill it with all the jars and tins of junk foods, refined sugars, and processed foods of all kinds. Give or throw the bag away immediately.

CHAPTER THIRTEEN: GET AMPLE SLEEP

The importance of ample sleep can never be underestimated in connection to binge eating. Here are some hidden connections between sleep and binge eating:

Some sufferers are so accustomed to sleep deprivation that they don't even mention it as a problem anymore unless they are asked the specific question by therapist(s). People with binge eating disorders who are sleep deprived are known to have one or more of these experiences:

- Their binge eating urges are stronger and more uncontrollable than normal cravings after dinner and before bedtime.
- They have almost insatiable cravings for highly palatable and processed foods filled with sugars, salts, and fats.
- Sleep-deprived people find it almost impossible to fight against their binge eating urges when they are fatigued.

These situations increase the difficulty for sleep-derived sufferers to fight against their disorder. Another common symptom with sufferers who have a problem with sleep is that they automatically turn to binge eating without even attempting self-care methods.

Here are some great tips to ensure you get sufficient sleep which, in turn, will help you manage binge eating better:

Ensure your sleep times are consistent – Decide what time you want to sleep and wake up each day. Adhere to this self-imposed sleep timetable even when you are not feeling sleepy. Avoid changing your sleep pattern during the weekends because your cycle will be disrupted even more than before. Stick to the predetermined time even on weekends.

If you haven't been able to sleep for about 10 minutes after you lie down on your bed, get off the bed, and try to read a book or magazine. Do not use mobiles, TVs, or any other electronic devices. Then, try and go back to sleep. Repeat this process until you fall asleep.

Identify the connection between sleep and your moods – Moods and feelings of anxiety play an important role in managing binge eating urges. When you feel depressed, your ability to ride the binge wave reduces considerably.

For people who struggle with mood swings, getting sufficient sleep is imperative. For this, you must identify how much your body and mind need rest to prevent the onset of bad moods. And stick to this duration of sleep irrespective of other issues.

Change your waking patterns – Often, people focus on getting to sleep at the right time and forget to watch their waking patterns. When the alarm rings in the morning, you must get off your bed. Pressing the 'snooze' button, and getting back to sleep for a few minutes more results in a shallow state of rest. Consequently, when the alarm rings at the end of the snooze period, you wake up feeling less fresh than you were when the alarm rang the first time. Each time you snooze, your sleep quality reduces, and you feel less fresh than the previous time. Instead, wake up at the first sound of the alarm, expose yourself to sunlight, get yourself a cup of coffee, and begin your day's work at an unhurried pace.

Today, before the end of the day, determine the most suitable time to go to bed and the perfect waking time for you. And stick to that from today onwards.

CHAPTER FOURTEEN: WHAT TO DO WHEN A BINGE COMES

Your journal entries will help you recognize signs and symptoms of an oncoming bingeing urge. Chapter Ten talks about the points to write down when you feel a bingeing urge coming on. Keep reading your journals so that you become familiar with the feelings and signs. Here are some tips on what you can do when a binge comes on:

Be mindful of the emotion – Identify the accompanying emotions, and sit quietly with them. Accept your feelings and urges without judging the emotions or yourself. Look at them without a feeling of right or wrong or about being vindicated or not. Just let them be.

Initially, this approach will be very hard because we are all trained and accustomed to reacting and responding to our feelings. However, when you consciously sit with your emotions and choose not to respond or react to them, you will notice that feelings reach a peak, and then simply disappear into oblivion. With patient and diligent practice, you will reach a situation when you will not need to binge to get rid of these emotions.

Ride the binge wave – Distract yourself with alternative options and ride the binge wave as you would surf the ocean waves. Your bingeing desire also has a limit on it. It cannot keep rising indefinitely. You need to find the resolve and wait for it to peak, and then the downturn will happen, and the urge will slowly but surely recede.

Of course, this approach is easier said than done. Writing it down, thinking about riding the wave, and actually experiencing the uncontrollable emotions are two different things. Yet, give yourself time and patience. Delay the binge each time, and your willpower and resolve will improve significantly. Here are some alternate distractions you can consider to ride the binge wave:

- Go outdoors for a walk
- Go play a favorite game
- Go to the park, and interact with other people
- Go for a long drive
- Mow the lawn or do some gardening
- Read a book
- Watch a movie
- Meditate
- Talk to someone you can trust

Chat with someone on a binge eating forum – Become a member of a binge eating forum. Most forums have 24/7 chat rooms where you could find other members going through the same problem as you are, and waiting to speak.

Go online, and speak to them. Also, there could be counselors who are available during that time. Use their services if you can. In whatever way you can, talking to somebody will help you pass the binge wave without much damage to your efforts.

Find your happy situation or place – Indulge in activities that make you feel good about yourself. Listen to a favorite song. If you play an instrument, then play your favorite song on it. Hit the gym. Go for a run or a walk. Watch a movie that makes you laugh. Avoid excessively emotional movies lest your binge urges get stronger than before.

As a first step toward applying the tips given in this chapter, reread your journal and identify repeated emotions that converge in your mind when a binge urge is coming on. Become familiar with these emotions.

CHAPTER FIFTEEN: TAKE THE POWER AWAY FROM FOOD

Remember that when you are binge eating, you are not in control of what is happening to you. Your food is controlling you. Taking power away from food is the step where you wrestle control back to yourself. You empower yourself to control food, and not accept things the other way around. Here are some steps to help you take away control and power from food:

List your binge foods – Again, use your journal to make a separate list of all the foods that you binge on. Against each of the food items, list out the negativities and health issues it can create. Look up the Internet, and write down the number of people affected by overconsumption of that particular food or some important ingredients in that food.

For example, excessive consumption of refined sugars is one of the biggest contributory factors for the increasing number of diabetes-affected people around the world. As per multiple statistics, nearly 30 million people in the US are affected by diabetes, and over 8 million people may not even be aware of the condition affecting their body! These staggering figures will wake your brain up and empower your willpower to fight against cravings for sugar-filled foods.

Here is another example to start a hate relationship with your favorite foods. Think of an image that disgusts you. It could be dead cockroaches or lizards or some other worm or insect. Now, picture these worms or insects that gross you out crawling out from your favorite pizza! Yuck!

You can rest assured this gross image will remain in your head for a long time, and could really help you keep away from pizza. Make sure you create as vivid an image as possible to ensure you are totally put off by the sight of that food.

Change the way your mind talks about food – If your thoughts are something like, "I feel deprived if I cannot have a couple of chocolate doughnuts now," change this thought too, "I feel so proud of myself that I am looking at these doughnuts, and can still walk away from them."

Change your self-narrative to positive stories. Compel your brain to convert negative thoughts into positive ones like the above example. Reframe limiting, negative self-talks to liberating, positive self-talk.

Give yourself non-food rewards – If you have managed to overcome a particular binge urge or even delayed the binge for a considerably long duration, then gift yourself with something that you have been wanting for a long time. It could be a small pair of earrings or a special book or a visit to the art gallery or some such thing. Primarily, through this approach, you are telling your brain that food is not the controller; you are, and it has to listen to your commands.

Don't deny yourself any foods – Avoid getting into diets that restrict intake of any kind of food. Your already anxious and stressed-out brain will get even more anxious at the thought of restrictions. And these limiting thoughts will fuel your bingeing urges even further. Therefore, don't deny yourself anything; simply remember to eat small portions of everything.

As a starter, create two positive thoughts to counter the following baseless negative ideas that keep creeping into the minds of most binge eating sufferers in some form or the other:

- I am a worthless person who has no control over my emotions.
- I wish I was never born.

CHAPTER SIXTEEN: BE MORE MINDFUL

Mindfulness is a beautiful concept that originated more than 2500 years ago in India when Lord Buddha preached it as a way to control and manage thoughts. Today, this concept has spread all over the world and an increasing number of people are taking advantage of its multiple benefits. It can be very useful in managing your binge eating urges.

So, what is mindfulness? Being mindful is being acutely aware of your feelings, thoughts, and your experiences in the present moment. Mindfulness is all about putting your entire being including your body, mind, and soul into this present moment instead of worrying about the past and/or the future.

With increasing mindfulness, you will find the power to be proud of and grateful for the many things you have achieved and the many things that you have received in your life. These positive thoughts help you counter negative thoughts, and with persistent practice, you will find yourself becoming increasingly adept at managing emotions maturely, and without the need for binge eating.

Compelling yourself to eat mindfully will help you eat slowly; a critical item to reduce bingeing. Here are some tips to cultivate mindfulness while eating.

Spend a few minutes on reflection before eating – Before you take your first bite, think about how you are feeling. Are you bored, stressed out, rushed, angry, sad, disappointed? Are you hungry or are you indulging in emotional eating? After a couple of minutes of reflection, you can choose to go ahead or back off from eating.

Sit down at the table – Don't eat while you are standing or walking. Sit at the table and eat. You will eat less if you avoid multitasking while eating. Also, turn off mobiles, TVs, and other distracting elements. Focus only on the food.

Serve out your food onto a plate – Don't eat directly from the tin or packet. Serve out the food onto a plate. If not for any other reason, the time taken to serve your food out could be used to reflect on your emotions and thoughts. Moreover, you are more likely to be conscious of your portion sizes when you see the food on your plate rather than dipping your hand or spoon or fork into the tin or packet.

Chew every bite at least 20 times – Yes, you must count the number of times you chew. Counting will make you focus on your chewing action, and you will slow down. Savor the bite in your mouth by focusing on its taste, texture and flavor. As you chew your food, try and identify the taste and/or the ingredients. Focusing on your mind on these elements will help you to not rush through your eating.

Prepare the next bite only after the previous bite is completely swallowed – Invariably, we are getting the next bite ready even when our mouth is full of food. Avoid this scenario. Instead, take your hand off the plate, and wait until your previous bite is completely swallowed. Then, reach out for your next bite.

Try and maintain silence during your meal – This tip will be easy to implement if you are binge eating because typically it happens in secret. Remain silent and bring the focus of your mind onto the eating and chewing action. The silence will help you appreciate your food, which is not what happens when you are binge eating as most of the time, you don't even know what you are consuming. Therefore, eating mindfully will help your brain be focused on the eating activity empowering you to be in control, and not the food.

Start being mindful by focusing on your thoughts and feelings that you are going through right now. Enter these thoughts into your journal right away.

CHAPTER SEVENTEEN: DAILY TRICKS TO HELP MANAGE BINGE-EATING

Here are some daily tricks and tips you can use to help prevent falling off the wagon.

Steer Clear of Diet Fads

Multiple studies have proven that when you are compelled to avoid certain types of food, your cravings and binge-eating urges increase. And all types of diets have some kinds of foods in their exclusion list.

Therefore, steer clear of all diet fads, and simply focus your entire attention on healthy small portions of healthy and nutritious foods of all kinds. You will have better control over your cravings.

Do Not Skip Meals

Skipping meals tends to increase your hunger pangs, which have a direct impact on cravings, which, in turn, could result in overeating. Studies have shown that eating one large meal each day instead of 3-4 small meals resulted in increased blood-sugar levels and the levels of ghrelin, the hunger-stimulating hormones.

Both these biological elements contribute significantly to binge-eating. Therefore, avoid skipping meals. Moreover, scientists have observed through various studies that people who start the day with a healthy, nutritious breakfast tend to have reduced ghrelin (the hunger-stimulating hormone) activity, which, in turn, results in lowered cravings.

Get Sufficient Sleep

Although this point has been made earlier too, it makes sense to include it in the daily tips because the lack of sleep has been directly connected to binge-eating as proven by many studies conducted by different experts in the medical field.

Eat Mindfully

When you eat slowly and mindfully, being aware of every emotion, feeling, taste, and other aspect of eating, you will be more aware of when you are feeling full which will help you stop eating. Mindful eating improves eating behaviors.

Get Physical Activity

Include a walk/run/gym regimen into your everyday routine. Many studies have revealed that binge-eating disorders are reduced significantly by increased physical activity. Additionally, physical activity has proven to enhance moods and reduce stress thereby preventing and/or decreasing emotional eating.

Drink Plenty of Water

Studies have proven that individuals who drinks plenty of water decreases their food consumption as compared to those who do not stay well-hydrated. Drinking water has been observed to boost metabolism and help in weight loss. Staying hydrated is critical to controlling your binge-eating behavior.

Include Plenty of Fiber in Your Daily Meals

Fiber reduces hunger pangs by moving slowly within the digestive tract, and also by keeping us feeling satiated for a sustained period of time. Scientific studies have shown increased fiber intake in daily meals reduces hunger pangs, calorie intake, and increases satiety.

Practice Yoga

Yoga is an ancient health-boosting technique that has exercises and postures designed to align and harmonize the workings of the body and mind. Studies have proven time and again that daily practice of yoga reduces cravings and helps you manage emotional eating problems.

Don't Forget to Update Your Journals

The importance of maintaining a journal for your binge-eating problem has already been stressed. Do not forget to update your food and mood journals on a daily basis. The entries made here will be the cornerstone of the success of your endeavor to get rid of the binge-eating disorder from your life.

Follow these daily tips and tricks unfailingly. Don't worry excessively about relapses. They are bound to happen. Get back on track and keep up your fight. Sustained victory has more to do with persistence and patient effort rather than occasional on and off blitzkrieg flashes.

CHAPTER EIGHTEEN: LONG-TERM BINGE EATING

Untreated and unresolved long-term binge eating can result in irreparable damage to your physical and mental systems. The risks of long-term binge eating include cardiovascular disease, high cholesterol, high blood pressure, arthritis, Type 2 diabetes, social isolation, depression and anxiety, and finally, loneliness to the point of becoming suicidal.

You have to start your treatment immediately. Visit your doctor first who will put you onto other medical professionals needed to treat your long-term binge eating disorder. You might need the help of a psychiatrist, psychologist, dietitian, family therapist, and a social worker who will all work in tandem to get faster and immediate relief that is absolutely essential to prevent the onset of such big health risks as mentioned above.

If you or any of your loved ones are repeatedly on this binge eating fix, they need help as early as possible. The tips and suggestions mentioned in this book will be useful too. However, the first line of treatment for long-term binge eaters has to necessarily come from qualified and trained professionals. They will need far more help than people who have dared to speak up and ask for help earlier.

The positive thing about binge eating disorders is that while long-term effects have big risks, the disorder itself can be managed and recovery can start no matter how deep an individual has fallen. The first step is to reach out for help. Then, the beginning of treatment itself might not be as difficult as that first step.

However, people recovering from long-term binge eating habits are at a higher risk of relapse than others. Therefore, it might be wise to have frequent counseling sessions during recovery to prevent relapses. Also, a loved one who can be with the affected individual right through the recovery process will prove to be very beneficial for the sufferer.

The first step is to seek help. Pick up that phone, and call someone you trust, or call the local therapist's helpline.

CHAPTER NINETEEN: MEN, DON'T FEEL ALONE

It is a common misconception that only women are victims to binge eating. Men can also be affected by this debilitating disorder. The extra burden on men is that in addition to all the other stigma that women sufferers are subjected to, they have to handle a condition that is wrongly considered to be a female-related one. This wrong misconception and the lack of sufficient knowledge enhances the difficulty for men.

However, if you are a guy struggling with binge eating disorder, you don't have to lose heart. Here are some things you can try out immediately:

- First, speak to your trusted general physician. Voice your concerns to him or her.
- Your doctor will put you on to psychologist or a psychiatrist who can help you arrive at the root cause of your binge eating problem which could be something to do with an unresolved mental issue or childhood trauma. If the problem goes deep, then your doctor could recommend medications to treat the unresolved hidden mental problems.
- Get the help of a dietician to find ways to change your eating habits for the better. Stick to a healthy diet, and find ways to get rid of junk from your vicinity.
- Get therapy to help you change your thoughts and feelings into positive ones. Take the tips given in this book, and start immediately.

- Accept and love yourself the way you are. Remember people across the world come in different shapes and sizes. There is nothing wrong with being different from others as long as you know what is healthy and unhealthy for you, and stay away from what's not good for you and embrace what's good for you.
- Do not forget to include physical activity in your daily routine.
- Learn to tune in to your body signals so that you can clearly discern between feeling full and feeling hungry.

Don't get into the mythical trap that binge eating disorders are a female thing. It can happen to anyone irrespective of gender, age, caste, creed, nationality, race, etc. Being a man does not mean hiding your fears under the carpet. It means finding the courage to ask for help. Asking for help is not a sign of weakness; it a sign of strength.

As a starting point, look within you and ask yourself if you are running away from the reality because you fear ridicule. If yes, change this thought, and don't allow insensitive people to take control of your life. Instead, you take control of your life and seek help.

CONCLUSION: THE BATTLE CONTINUES

The biggest lesson about your binge-eating habit is to learn that the disorder pretends to help you by making you think you are in control because of your relationship with food and craving. But, in reality, it is controlling you because the binge-eating habit makes you forget about the rest of the world around you; your family, your loved ones, your friends, and your entire life.

The binge-eating habit is like a manipulative parasite that seems to convince you that without it, you don't have an identity. It is up to you to wrestle control of your life from this parasitic disease so that you can achieve what you are born for.

Once you take back the control of your life into your own hands, the war cry is sounded. Then, this debilitating habit starts to use various defensive and offensive modes to take back control of your life. And each battle you win against this horrible habit will make you stronger than before ensuring the next battle is less difficult.

But, you can rest assured the battle will continue for some time, and you will have to delve deeply into your mind to harness every ounce of the reserves of your willpower and mental strength to win it. Remember, your willpower and mental stress are similar to muscles, the more you work them, the stronger they get.

Yes, your journey is not going to be a smooth upward-moving graph. It is going to be a spiral when some days are going to be so bad that you want to simply forget everything, and get back to your habit. The trick is to recognize these down times and keep motivating yourself and not give up. The relapses will happen, and each time you get up to fight against the relapse, your strength to fight against binge-eating urges will improve.

So, don't give up even if you seem to fall off the wagon. Get back up, and continue your battle. You are bound to see victory sooner than later.

Don't forget the importance of self-love and self-compassion. Love yourself for who you are, and be proud of whatever you have achieved in your life. People who give negative criticism are usually those who lack self-confidence and use nastiness to reflect their true personalities. Keep such people away from your life, and just focus on improving yourself.

Remember to treat yourself as you would treat an adorable child. Respect and love yourself for who and what you are. Don't focus entirely on your binge eating disorder. Focus on your strengths and powers as well. Make it your purpose to feel emotionally secure, and that is when you will be empowered to fight your continued battles with binge eating.

USEFUL INFORMATION

Here are some useful links to organizations that help sufferers of binge eating disorders:

https://www.beateatingdisorders.org.uk/types/binge-eating-disorder - You can read up a lot more about binge eating disorders. You have support services, recovery services, and lot more on offer here. You can interact with other sufferers and take solace in the fact that you are not alone.

https://www.nationaleatingdisorders.org/learn/by-eating-disorder/bed - While the above organization is BEAT in UK, this link is for NEDA in the US. Here too, you can reach out to professionals and sufferers and get all kinds of help regarding binge eating disorders.

Here are a couple more forums for you:

https://www.nhs.uk/Conditions/Binge-eating/Pages/community.aspx

https://www.eatingdisorder.org/forum/

RESOURCES

https://www.youtube.com/watch?v=STkBb9mo0fQ

https://www.youtube.com/watch?v=TS09i1OZzWY

https://www.youtube.com/watch?v=cyH2kEWuVRo

https://www.youtube.com/watch?v=lzqKZ2fCAHQ

https://www.healthline.com/nutrition/how-to-stop-binge-eating#section1

https://www.nhs.uk/conditions/binge-eating/treatment/

https://www.independent.co.uk/life-style/health-and-families/binge-eating-how-to-stop-overeating-emotional-tips-nutritionist-jessica-sepel-a8318081.html

https://www.beateatingdisorders.org.uk/types/binge-eating-disorder

https://www.nationaleatingdisorders.org/i-cant-stop-binge-eating-and-it-beginning-consume-my-life

https://www.sane.org/the-sane-blog/my-story/reflecting-on-my-binge-eating-disorder

https://www.healthline.com/nutrition/common-eating-disorders#section9

https://www.helpguide.org/articles/diets/emotional-eating.htm

https://www.beateatingdisorders.org.uk/

https://greatist.com/happiness/science-why-we-binge https://www.waldeneatingdisorders.com/8-myths-about-binge-eating-disorder/ https://www.jackcanfield.com/blog/how-to-create-an-empowering-vision-book/ https://www.fightbingeeating.com/blog/5-ways-using-bullet-journal-emotional-eating

https://www.webmd.com/mental-health/eating-disorders/binge-eating-disorder/binge-eating-disorder-men#2

www.ingramcontent.com/pod-product-compliance
Lightning Source LLC
Chambersburg PA
CBHW070035040426
42333CB00040B/1682